NEVER PMS AGAIN

KAMILI KIONGOZI

ISBN: 9798662964877

Cover design by: Kamili Kiongozi
Icon made by Freepik from www.flaticon.com
Printed in the United States of America

This publication is designed to provide accurate and authoritative information in regard to the subject matter covered. It is sold with the understanding that neither the author nor the publisher is engaged in rendering medical services or other professional services. The information in this book should not take the place of medical advice. If medical advice or other expert assistance is required, the services of a competent professional person should be sought.

TABLE OF CONTENTS

CONTENTS

Congrats on taking the first step to making a change in your life! I used to be like you – glad to be a woman, but decidedly *not* glad about suffering every month!

I learned about menstruation at age 10, and after that, I absolutely dreaded getting my period. When I got my first period at age 14, I was devastated – the dreaded plight had finally befallen me! My mother did her best to help me see that menstruation wasn't terrible, but just a part of becoming a woman. That was all fine and dandy, until summertime came, and I couldn't go swimming due to my period! Oh, I spent years feeling like my period ruined my life once a month. Then, around age 25, I started experiencing PMS. I *really* hated my period then! It wasn't fair that I was forced against my will to suffer *and* bleed!

My suffering began with my skin – I used to have beautiful, flawless skin. But then, I started breaking out every single month. The acne bumps wouldn't last that long, but they left scars. My lower back hurt. I would get extremely hot for no apparent reason. My emotions were all over the place. I was inexplicably tired. My breasts would get extremely sore and tender. In short, I was miserable! Some of you have had similar symptoms, and many of you have suffered much worse.

Like you, I finally decided that a change had to be made. I am now free of PMS completely! It's been many years since I last suffered due to my menstrual cycle. In this book, I will tell you exactly what I learned, what I did, and how you too can never suffer from PMS again.

On my personal journey, I consulted with doctors and nutritionists to find the root cause of my problem and solve it. This book will use a science-based approach to provide information about PMS and its root cause, as well as give you a step-by-step guide to tackle that root cause and avoid PMS forever.

I'll tell you up front – for many of you, this will not be easy. If you follow the method described in this book, results will be seen immediately; however, becoming free from PMS will require work, self-discipline, and commitment. You will more than likely have to make big changes in your life. But don't get discouraged! By the end of this book, I guarantee that you will have all of the knowledge and tools you need to lead a better life free from PMS.

What is PMS?

First of all, let's talk about what PMS is *not*. PMS is not a disease or a medical condition. PMS is not an excuse to be in a bad mood when you're on your period. PMS is not a design flaw in women. PMS is not some kind of curse on women.

PMS stands for **P**re-**M**enstrual **S**yndrome. "Pre" means "before" and of course "menstrual" means your "menstrual cycle," or your period. "Syndrome" is "a combination of symptoms resulting from a single cause or so commonly occurring together as to constitute a distinct clinical picture." So, in simple terms, PMS is the group of symptoms that are all caused by the same thing that we experience *before* our menstrual cycle.

WHAT ARE SOME SIGNS OF PMS?

Most of you already know the answer to this! Remember, PMS is a <u>group</u> of symptoms. All women's bodies are special and unique, and you may experience any number of these symptoms:

Physical symptoms:

- Headaches

- Cramping

- Swollen hands and feet

- Feeling bloated around your stomach

- Sore, swollen, and/or tender breasts

- Muscle aches

- Joint pain

- Hunger (yes, those cravings are probably due to PMS!)

- Fatigue
- Changes in bowel movements (for some of you it's extra poos, for some of you it's no poos at all!)
- Acne and skin breakouts, usually along your jaw line

Emotional/mental symptoms:
- Mood swings
- Irritability or hostile behavior
- Feeling tired
- Sleep problems (sleeping too much or too little)
- Trouble with concentration or memory
- Tension or anxiety
- Depression, feelings of sadness, or crying spells
- Changes in libido

Women's bodies are always changing, so you may have experienced different symptoms at different points in your life. For example, when I was in my early 20s, I experienced lower back aches only occasionally, and no other symptoms. In my late 20s, the back pain worsened and became more frequent, and I started experiencing acne breakouts, mood swings, and tender breasts. I've had no PMS in my 30s though!

Another indicator of PMS is timing. Remember that PMS is *pre*-menstrual. This means that PMS symptoms occur *before* your period. If you experience any of these symptoms after the first day or two of your menstruation, or after your menstrual cycle, then it is not due to PMS.

WHAT CAUSES PMS?

To understand PMS and its causes, we need to understand what's happening in our menstrual cycle before the menstruation phase (again, <u>pre</u>-menstrual). Menstrual cycles have four phases:

1) Menstrual phase – This is when you have your period. During this time, you shed the thickened lining of your uterus wall. This phase usually lasts 3-8 days.

2) Follicular phase – This phase begins on the same day as the Menstrual phase and ends when ovulation occurs. During this phase, which usually lasts 10-16 days, a new egg will mature and your uterus lining will begin to thicken.

3) Ovulation phase – This phase is when your ovaries release the egg that matured in the Follicular phase. This phase only lasts for 24 hours. During this phase, a mature egg will either be fertilized, and you'll become pregnant, or it will not fertilize and will dissolve.

4) Luteal phase – This phase is the time span between ovulation and menstruation, and usually lasts 14 days. During this time, your uterine walls will grow thicker. If you've become pregnant, the uterine wall thickness will protect the fetus. If you are not pregnant, then you'll cycle back to the Menstrual phase and shed the uterus wall lining during your period.

Our hormone production changes throughout the month as we go through each phase of our menstrual cycle. During each phase, your body produces a different amount of estrogen, progesterone, serotonin, and eicosanoids. These levels vary from woman to woman, but your body requires a certain ratio to be maintained. Maintaining these ratios is called hormonal balance. However, if your body produces much more or much less of any of those hormones, then the ratio will not be maintained, and the result will be a hormonal imbalance.

Hormonal imbalances can cause various problems depending on the menstrual phase in which they occur. Pre-Menstrual Syndrome is the result of a hormonal imbalance that occurs during the last half of the luteal phase. Every month during the luteal phase of your menstrual cycle, progesterone levels will rise for 7 days, and then decrease for 7 days. During those final 7 days when progesterone is naturally decreasing, any disruption in the ratio of estrogen, progesterone, serotonin, and eicosanoids will cause a hormonal imbalance. That hormonal imbalance is the root cause of the group of symptoms described as Pre-Menstrual Syndrome.

Dr. Anna Cabeca, author of "The Hormone Fix," states it succinctly: "Starting our periods and ending our periods is mandatory. That's a life cycle — but suffering and [being] symptomatic is optional, and that's a function of hormonal imbalance, whether we're in our teens or in perimenopause or menopause age range." PMS is not a disease nor a requirement of womanhood. Pharmaceutical companies construct entire marketing campaigns to convince women that we are all born with some kind of flaw resulting in a chronic disease that requires prescription medication. This is simply false. PMS is NOT natural or necessary, neither does it require medication. It is simply the result of a hormonal imbalance.

I chose to opt out of suffering and being symptomatic, and you can too. In the coming chapters, I will share with you an action-oriented plan so that you too can live a life free from PMS.

CHAPTER 2

How can I prevent PMS?

There is no cure per se for PMS. Since PMS is caused by a hormonal imbalance during the week prior to your menstruation, the solution to preventing PMS is to balance your hormones in that week.

STEP 1: TRACK YOUR MENSTRUAL CYCLE

PMS <u>only</u> occurs in the last half of the luteal phase. This is the 7 days leading up to your period. For example, if your period is scheduled to begin on the 8th of the month, then you may experience PMS starting from the 1st of the month.

If you have no idea when your next period is coming, or if you only have a vague idea, then you won't know when that 7-day PMS time span is, and you won't be able to balance your hormones when they need balancing. This is why tracking your menstrual cycle is the first step to preventing PMS. There are plenty of apps that help you track your period, and any one of them will do. However, we need to track our periods and the seven days before it, so I recommend using a calendar or a planner.

HOW TO TRACK YOUR PERIOD

A woman's menstrual cycle will occur every X amount of days. On average, a woman's cycle occurs every 28 days, but it can be anywhere from 21 to 45 days. Whatever it is for you, it will be an exact number. So if you menstruate in a 28-day cycle, your period will not come *approximately* every 28 days, it will always come *exactly* every 28 days.

To track your period, you need to know the exact days of two periods. For example, let's say that today is May 29th and my period began today. Let's also say that my last period began on May 1st. From this, I know how long my cycle is – 28 days. Now that I know the length of my cycle, I can accurately predict the exact date of my next period:

(Last menstrual start date) + (cycle length) = Next menstrual start date

Our example: May 29th + 28 days = June 26

So let's get started!

If you have already been tracking your period: Great! Mark your calendar or your planner for your next Menstrual Start Date. Then go back seven days and mark that entire 7-day time span as Pre-Menstrual. Step 1 done! Treat yourself to something nice for being on top of things!

If you have not been tracking your period, but have a

vague idea when your last one began: That's ok! For example, if you think to yourself "hm I recall my last period came about two weeks ago," then mark in your calendar two weeks ago from today. Then, use that date to predict your next period. Remember that menstrual cycles are an exact science, so if your period did NOT come two weeks ago from today, but actually came two weeks ago from yesterday, then your prediction for your next period will be off by one day. That's ok! Go ahead and mark in your planner or calendar your Estimated Menstrual Start Date. Then go back seven days and mark that entire 7-day time span as Estimated Pre-Menstrual. Step 1 done! Once your next period comes, then you'll know the length of your cycle and you'll be able to predict the exact date of your Menstrual Start Date and Pre-Menstrual Week. Treat yourself to something nice for being a Great Guesstimator! (It's a real thing).

If you have not been tracking your period and have no clue when it's coming: Living life on the edge! Reminds me of a younger, more spontaneous me! In this case, I recommend waiting until your next period comes and then marking your calendar. Feel free to treat yourself to something nice because why not?

Tracking your menstrual cycle is an exact science. However, there are a few things that can throw off this rhythm. You may have heard that women's periods will align when they are together. This is not a myth! If you start spending a significant amount of time around a different group of women, then either your period will change its timing, their periods will change timing, or all of your periods will change timing. For example, you might get a new female roommate, or new female coworkers, or join a convent. Doctors and researchers have not discovered why this happens, but they are sure that it does indeed happen. If you start spending a significant amount of time around new adult females, you should lookout for changes in the timing of your period.

STEP 2: BALANCE YOUR HORMONES

Ok! Now that you've marked your Menstrual Start Date and your Pre-Menstrual week, you'll know exactly when your hormones need to be balanced. So let's get into what you should do to balance your hormones.

There are three factors that are causing you to have a hormonal imbalance and suffer from PMS. In the coming chapters, I will elaborate on each of these and give you specific actions to take:

1) Diet - This is the most important part of your Pre-Menstrual week. If you are experiencing PMS, I guarantee that it's mostly caused from your diet. You are what you eat, and what you eat can either balance your hormones or throw them out of whack. There are specific foods that cause hormonal imbalance. Cutting out those foods during your PMS week will help to balance your hormones. There are also certain nutrients that you should intake during your PMS week to help balance your hormones. These are not diet-specific – you can get these nutrients whether you have specific dietary restrictions or not. In Chapters 3 and 4, I'll give you information about which foods to avoid and which foods to eat in order to balance your hormones.

2) Exercise - Exercising has been proven to affect hormone production and regulation. Don't worry, you don't need to join a gym! In Chapter 5, I will discuss how you can use exercise to help regulate and balance your hormones.

3) Lifestyle - There are additional lifestyle factors that you can change and improve during your Pre-Menstrual week to help balance your hormones. I'll cover these in Chapter 6.

The only way to guarantee results is to change your lifestyle to incorporate all three of these changes. You might see results if you *only* make dietary changes or *only* exercise or *only* make lifestyle changes. However, all of these factors are unbalancing your hormones, so if you don't address all of them, then your hormones will still be unbalanced and you may continue to suffer from PMS.

GETTING INTO THE RIGHT MINDSET

Before we move forward to the step-by-step details, I

want you to take this time to re-adjust your mindset. Most of us have been conditioned to think of our menstrual cycle as a hindrance, and to think of PMS as a terrible yet unavoidable part of womanhood. None of those things are true. PMS is completely avoidable! As I wrote in the introduction, what I'm going to share with you in the coming chapters will require you to change your life. You can look at this as a sacrifice, just another part of the plight of womanhood, but that's a negative, glass-half-empty view. Womanhood is not a plight. I took that negative view when I first began managing my PMS symptoms. I felt that I needed to sacrifice to achieve my goal, and that's what everything felt like – an unfair sacrifice. If you take that view, then getting rid of PMS will be *extremely* difficult for you. At every turn, you'll feel like you're choosing between a rock and a hard place.

Changing your mindset can change your life. There is plenty of evidence that this is true – in his book "The 7 Habits of Highly Effective People," Stephen R. Covey talks about how a change in your mindset produces a change in results. The power of the mind is also a common theme in metaphysics. After successfully making changes, becoming PMS-free, and seeing how my entire life improved, I began to take a glass-half-full view. I realized that my PMS week wasn't a week of sacrifice. The week before my period was one week that I took every single month to take supreme care of my physical and mental health, and I began looking at it as week of self-care.

If you're reading this book, then clearly you want something to change in your life. I encourage you to first change your mindset about your menstrual cycle. For the rest of this book, I will refer to the week before your period as your PMSC Week – your **P**re-**M**enstrual **S**elf-**C**are Week.

Ready to change your life and be free of PMS forever? Let's do it!

CHAPTER 3

Eating for Hormonal Balance: Foods to Avoid

Dr. Christiane Northrup writes "The standard American diet almost guarantees some kind of hormone imbalance [in women] because it is high in simple (or refined) sugars and starches, the wrong kinds of fats, and low-fiber, nutrient-poor fast foods." To balance your hormones through dietary changes requires doing two things: 1) avoiding foods that unbalance your hormones, and 2) adding foods that help to balance your hormones. This chapter will cover the foods that cause a hormone imbalance.

AVOIDING FOODS THAT UNBALANCE YOUR HORMONES

There are seven foods that you should completely avoid during your Pre-Menstrual Self-Care Week. These foods all cause a hormone imbalance, and to prevent suffering from PMS, you should omit all of these foods from your diet during your PMSC Week when your hormone production levels are changing.

1) NO alcohol

No drinking during your Pre-Menstrual Self-Care Week. No glass of wine after work, no beer with your turkey burger, no mimosa at brunch.

Alcohol affects your hormones because it significantly interferes with estrogen metabolism. It causes an almost immediate hormonal imbalance, with too much estrogen in the blood relative to progesterone.

Sugar and caffeine are also on our list, so you can't

replace an alcoholic drink with soda or mocktails. Take this week to stay hydrated and drink water or juice. For a cocktail replacement, mix sparkling water with juice.

2) NO caffeine

No coffee, no black or green tea, no energy drinks, no caffeinated beverages.

It's well-established that caffeine contributes to estrogen dominance, which can mean one of two things: we either have too much estrogen in relation to progesterone, or we have an imbalance in the estrogen metabolites. Either way, that's a hormonal imbalance and will cause PMS. In addition, studies have shown that caffeine increases cortisol and epinephrine while at rest, and that after caffeine consumption, levels of cortisol are similar to those experienced during acute stress. This means that caffeine re-creates stress conditions for the body. We'll get to stress in Chapter 6, but for now just know this – stress also causes a hormonal imbalance.

Caffeine can be replaced with naturally invigorating teas, such as peppermint. In Chapter 6, I will discuss lifestyle changes that you should make during your PMSC Week, one of which is getting sufficient sleep. If you make time to get a good night's sleep every night this week, you may find that you won't feel the need to consume caffeine.

Note: If this one will be a struggle for you, as it was/is for me, it may be helpful to start out by reducing your caffeine intake. Switching from coffee to black or green tea, or cutting back from 3-4 cups of coffee per day to just one cup will reduce your caffeine consumption. Keep in mind though, caffeine causes a hormonal imbalance, so you may still experience PMS symptoms if you only reduce your caffeine intake.

3) NO salt

No garlic salt, no seasoning salt, no Himalayan pink salt. Do not sprinkle salt on anything. Do not use it to season your food when cooking. Do not buy food that has high salt content.

Sodium naturally tends to decrease in the luteal phase of your menstrual cycle. The hormone that affects sodium balance is progesterone. Consuming additional salt during your PMSC Week affects your sodium balance, which in turn affects your hormonal balance. Have your PMS symptoms ever included bloating or puffiness? That's due to salt, which can cause bloating and water retention. Omitting, or seriously reducing, your salt intake will help you avoid bloating and help to maintain hormonal balance.

When cooking, replace salt with seasoning powders like onion powder, garlic powder, paprika, lemon pepper, etc. Personally, there are certain foods that I feel require salt to be delicious, like french fries and popcorn. So during my PMSC week, I simply avoid foods that I feel truly need salt.

Note: Quite a lot of finished food products have salt in them, like condiments or bread. In my experience, the tiny amount of added salt in your ketchup will not ruin your plan to never PMS again.

4) NO processed or refined sugar

Refined sugar is sugar that has been processed, as opposed to the natural sugars found in foods like fruit, for example. The most common refined sugar is table sugar, or sucrose, but there are also powdered sugars, syrups, and natural processed sugars. During your Pre-Menstrual Self-Care Week, completely omit foods and beverages that include sugar. No candy, no cake, no soft drinks, no desserts. No adding sugar to your caffeine-free tea.

When we eat sugar, including foods that convert to sugar (like carbohydrates), insulin is released to balance blood sugar by managing where and how glucose is stored in the body. This hormonal response is great for managing the occasional natural sugar (think fruits) or complex carb (think pasta), but when faced with a diet high in these foods (like the standard American diet), the body is forced to overproduce insulin in an effort to keep blood sugar balanced. As this is happening, your body is focusing more on insulin and processing the sugar, causing an imbalance with other hormones such as cortisol, progesterone, estrogen, and testosterone. A prolonged high-sugar diet can result in insulin resistance due to the constant overproduction of insulin. Consistently having too much insulin in the bloodstream results in negative health effects like diabetes, and will also have a negative effect on your hormonal balance.

Refined sugar can be substituted with sugar-free sweeteners like Stevia, coconut palm sugar, blackstrap molasses, and organic honey (don't get honey with added sugar! Kind of defeats the purpose. If you've never had real honey, you'll thank me).

Note: Like salt, quite a lot of finished food products have added sugar, high-fructose corn syrup, or some other variation of refined sugar. This is bad for your health, and in general, you should work to remove these harmful ingredients from your diet. For most of us though, it won't ruin our plan to never suffer from PMS again. Focus on cutting out food items with high sugar content like desserts, soft drinks, and processed foods, and you'll see results.

5) NO red meat

"Red meat" generally refers to meat that stays red after it's been cooked. "Red meat" also refers to meats with a nutritional content that is comparable to beef. Red meats include beef, lamb, pork, and goat, as well as "gamey" meats like deer, boar, and hare.

200 years ago, there was nothing really wrong with red meat. Today, however, there are seven hormones (testosterone propionate, trenbolone acetate, estradiol, zeranol, progesterone, melengestrol acetate, and bovine somatotropin) that are used in the commercial production of meat, eggs, and dairy products that wreak havoc on estrogen levels in humans. This means that the hormones and antibiotics in commercially raised cattle and poultry imbalance the ratio of estrogen and progesterone. This is especially true for red meat. Many countries, and the EU, ban imports of American beef due to concerns over these hormones. In addition, red meat is typically higher in saturated fats, which are the bad kind of fats that cause heart problems, cancer, and weight gain. So removing red meats from your diet, even for only one week every month, will not only prevent PMS, but will also improve your overall health.

During your PMSC week, if you are a meat-eater, you should completely avoid red meat and eat only "white meats," which include poultry, such as chicken and turkey, and seafood. Ideally, you should avoid all industrially-produced meat during this week and eat only wild-caught white meat and seafood.

6) NO dairy

No half-and-half with your non-caffeinated beverages. No cheese on your sandwich. No yogurt, eggs, or butter. No prepackaged dairy beverages.

Dairy disrupts hormonal balance in many ways – it can be irritating to the gut; it can be inflammatory; and, as mentioned above in the "NO red meat" section, the commercial production of dairy contains hormones and antibiotics that ruin your hormonal balance.

There are plenty of product substitutions that are readily available for purchase online or in your local grocery store. For example, cow's milk can be substituted with plant-based milk. I recommend substituting with oat milk – it has a consistency similar to cow's milk, has a very neutral taste, so it doesn't change the flavor of your food or beverages, and it's full of vitamins and nutrients. Butter can be substituted with healthy oils like olive oil or grapeseed oil.

7) NO processed foods

A processed food is any food that has been altered in some way during preparation. Food processing includes pasteurizing, freezing, fermenting, packaging, baking, drying, adding ingredients to extend shelf life, and more.

Most of the food available in grocery stores today is processed to at least some degree, but not all processed food is created equal. Some foods require processing to make them safe, such as orange juice, which needs to be pasteurized to remove harmful bacteria. Minimal processing cleans food, preserves it, or removes inedible parts, and keeps the nutritional content of the food pretty much the same. Examples of minimally processed foods are whole-grain flours and pastas, and coffee beans. However, chemically processed foods, also called ultra-processed foods, tend to be high in sugar, artificial ingredients, refined carbohydrates, and trans fats, all of which disrupt your hormonal balance.

During your Pre-Menstrual Self-Care Week, you should avoid chemically processed foods and anything with artificial ingredients such as fast food, junk food, ready-made snacks (candy, cookies, chips, etc), luncheon meats, sugary cereals, and microwavable meals.

PMS PREVENTION MEAL PLANNING

Some of you are saying to yourselves right now "I can't cut out all those foods! What will I eat?!" Relax, there are so many meal options! Baked salmon (or tofu) with rice and veggies, jerk chicken (or tofu) with rice and beans, and bbq chicken (or tofu) with corn and collard greens are just a few examples of meals that don't include any of the hormone-imbalancing foods above. To make things easier for yourself, I recommend planning all your meals during your PMSC Week to ensure that you easily avoid consuming foods that throw your hormones out of whack.

If you don't like to cook, or don't have the time, you can still avoid the foods that unbalance your hormones. You can order jerk chicken with plantain and rice and peas from your local Jamaican restaurant. You can order fish tacos with rice and beans (no cheese or sour cream!) from your local Mexican restaurant. You can order chicken pad thai (no egg!) from your local Thai restaurant. You can order chicken pasta with tomato sauce, or vegetable pasta from your local Italian restaurant. Unfortunately, most American cultural foods are bad for your health, and they should be avoided during your PMSC Week. Ordering food is not an ideal solution because it's impossible to completely avoid salt, sugar, and processed foods when a restaurant is making the preparations. You will experience a reduction of symptoms, but you may not be able to completely avoid PMS if your diet is mostly met by ordering out. Even if you order out, I still recommend you plan your meals during your Pre-Menstrual Self-Care Week.

SETTING YOURSELF UP FOR SUCCESS

It's important to make this as easy for yourself as possible. Some of the foods above will be easy for you to cut out, but we all have a food weakness. For me, cutting out sugar and caffeine was the hardest part of this hormone-balancing dietary regimen. I love sweet foods and desserts! I'm originally from the South, where we have the best desserts, but they are all full of refined sugar, salt, and dairy, and are usually highly processed – all things that should be avoided during the PMSC Week! I'll be honest – sometimes I still struggle with avoiding refined sugar (how much damage can one Krispy Kreme donut do, right?!). I tried (unsuccessfully) to substitute delicious desserts with all-natural, dairy-free, sugar-free desserts. I tried (also unsuccessfully) to substitute my morning coffee with iron-rich beverages. I found that for me, it's better to just go without, than to disappoint myself and disrespect my taste buds.

I know that my food weakness is caffeine and sugar, I know that I don't like substitutions, and I know that it's difficult to fight against cravings. Knowing those facts, each month I take steps to set myself up for success by preemptively avoiding the desires in the first place. To help curb my desire for caffeine, I make sure to get more than enough sleep each night. Therefore, I'm unlikely to feel a need for coffee to get through the day. I found that my cravings for sweets are strongest when I'm hungry. Instead of trying to ignore the cravings, which is difficult for me, I preemptively curb my desire for sweets by munching on fruits and nuts between meals.

One of the symptoms of PMS is cravings. In fact, unbalanced hormones can cause you to have cravings for unhealthy food specifically. Once you start balancing your hormones, it'll be easier to avoid the foods that throw your hormones out of balance. In the meantime, identify your food weakness and preemptively help yourself avoid it

For meal plan suggestions to help you stick to this hormone-balancing dietary regimen, please see Appendix III. Fear not ladies, you CAN do it! For some of you it will be difficult, but trust me, seven days of cutting out these foods will do *wonders* for your life!

CHAPTER 4

Eating for Hormonal Balance: Adding Omega-3s

In Western societies, consumption of omega-3 fatty acids has decreased dramatically over the past 150 years. Omega-3 deficiency directly causes hormone imbalance, and adding them to your diet immediately works to balance your hormones. This entire chapter is dedicated to omega-3 fatty acids, because they are just that important, and will literally change your life!

WHAT ARE OMEGA-3 FATTY ACIDS?

Omega-3 fatty acids (omega-3s) are a type of polyunsaturated fatty acids. There are eleven different types of omega-3s, and they all have slightly different roles in the body. The majority of scientific research, however, focuses on the three most important: alpha-linolenic acid (ALA), eicosapentaenoic acid (EPA), and docosahexaenoic acid (DHA). ALA is considered an essential fatty acid, which means it must be obtained from your diet. ALA can be converted into EPA and then to DHA, but the conversion is very limited. Therefore, EPA and DHA should also be consumed directly from foods and/or dietary supplements in order to increase levels of these fatty acids in the body.

But enough of the scientific mumbo jumbo! What does all this mean? Basically it means that you should eat foods that are high in ALA, EPA, and DHA omega-3s. These omega-3s can be easily found in a variety of foods, like certain nuts and seeds, fatty fish, and leafy green vegetables. More on sources of omega-3s later.

HOW DOES OMEGA-3 CONSUMPTION AFFECT PMS?

Omega-3s supply the necessary building blocks for hormone production and function. Deficiencies in omega-3s are directly responsible for imbalanced eicosanoids and overproduction of estrogen. That's right – your lack of omega-3s is one of the major factors throwing your hormones out of whack and causing your PMS!

Adding omega-3s to your diet will help to regulate estrogenic production and activity, and will also reduce inflammation, which exacerbates PMS symptoms. A diet supplemented with omega-3s fats has been shown to alleviate conditions associated with eicosanoid imbalance, including PMS, eczema, breast tenderness, acne, brittle fingernails, psoriasis, and dry skin. Foods that are high in omega-3 fatty acids will support hormone balance, which is exactly what you need for your PMSC Week. For that reason, adding omega-3s to your diet is equally as important as removing hormone-imbalancing foods from your diet.

HOW CAN I ADD OMEGA-3 FATTY ACIDS TO MY DIET?

Food Sources - Omega-3 fatty acids are found naturally in a variety of foods. Below I've listed the sources with the highest omega-3 content:

<u>ALA Sources:</u>

- Seeds – camelina seeds, chia seeds, flaxseed, hemp seeds, kiwifruit seeds, lingonberry seeds, perilla (also called shiso or kkaennip) seeds, pumpkin seeds, sea buckthorn, walnuts
- Plant oils – algae oil, camelina seed oil, canola oil (also called rapeseed oil), flaxseed oil, hemp oil, lingonberry seed oil, perilla oil, soybean oil, wheat germ oil

<u>EPA & DHA Sources:</u>

- Fatty cold water fish – herring, mackerel, salmon, sardines, tuna
- Marine meats – mussels, oysters
- Marine plants – algae
- Food brands of eggs, yogurt, juices, milk, and soy

beverages that are fortified with DHA and other omega-3s

Supplements - Omega-3 fatty acids can be taken in capsules as over-the-counter supplements or prescription medication. Over-the-counter supplements will specify the type of omega-3s in their ingredients. You can find these supplements in your local grocery store, health food store, vitamin or supplement store, or online:

- Algae Oil Supplements (often marketed as vegan omega-3s, or plant-based alternatives to fish oil supplements)
- Cod Liver Oil Supplements
- Fish Oil Supplements
- Flaxseed Oil Supplements
- Krill Oil Supplements
- Omega-3 Supplements

Medical studies conducted in the United Kingdom and Australasia demonstrate high-level evidence that omega-3 supplements lack efficacy across a range of health outcomes for which their use is advocated. In addition, the US federal government's 2015-2020 Dietary Guidelines for Americans notes that "nutritional needs should be met primarily from foods." Therefore, I recommend getting omega-3s from food sources rather than from supplements. Getting omega-3s from food sources is effective, can be modified to suit your body and lifestyle specifically, and has no side effects – don't like canola oil? No worries, use soybean oil instead. Kids don't like salmon dinners? Make tuna. Don't eat meat? Eat flax or chia seeds.

Keep in mind that your Pre-Menstrual Self-Care Week is all about what is best for <u>you</u> and <u>your</u> lifestyle. Again, I recommend increasing your intake of omega-3s from food sources, but both the USDA and the American FDA recommend dietary supplements for Americans who are unwilling or unable to get sufficient nutrition from food sources. Perhaps you live in a food desert, or don't enjoy cooking, or are responsible for feeding multiple people who aren't interested in their health. Maybe your local grocer doesn't carry flax seeds or any cold water fish. Or maybe you just enjoy the ease and simplicity of taking one capsule daily. Getting omega-3s from food sources is ideal and proven to work, but there is evidence that supplements could also be effective.

HOW MUCH OMEGA-3S DO I NEED TO CONSUME?

The National Academy of Medicine has provided an index for the Adequate Intake (AI) of omega-3s. Women ages 14+ should consume at least 1.1 grams (1,100 mg or 0.4 oz or approximately 3/4 tablespoons) of ALA omega-3 fatty acids daily. Foods with ALA omega-3s are the most important to consume during your PMSC Week. The National Academy of Medicine has not provided any Adequate Intake guidelines for EPA or DHA omega-3s, but most experts recommend a daily dosage of 1,000 mg of EPA and DHA combined.

Please see Table 2 on page 44 for a list of foods and their amount of ALA omega-3 fatty acids per serving, provided by the USDA.

For meat-eaters, I recommend eating fatty cold-water

Food	Grams / serving		
	ALA	DHA	EPA
Flaxseed oil, 1 tbsp	7.26		
Chia seeds, 1 ounce	5.06		
English walnuts, 1 ounce	2.57		
Flaxseed, whole, 1 tbsp	2.35		
Salmon, Atlantic, farmed cooked, 3 ounces		1.24	0.59
Salmon, Atlantic, wild, cooked, 3 ounces		1.22	0.35
Herring, Atlantic, cooked, 3 ounces*		0.94	0.77
Canola oil, 1 tbsp	1.28		
Sardines, canned in tomato sauce, drained, 3 ounces*		0.74	0.45
Mackerel, Atlantic, cooked, 3 ounces*		0.59	0.43
Salmon, pink, canned, drained, 3 ounces*	0.04	0.63	0.28
Soybean oil, 1 tbsp	0.92		
Trout, rainbow, wild, cooked, 3 ounces		0.44	0.4
Black walnuts, 1 ounce	0.76		
Mayonnaise, 1 tbsp	0.74		
Oysters, eastern, wild, cooked, 3 ounces	0.14	0.23	0.3
Sea bass, cooked, 3 ounces*		0.47	0.18
Edamame, frozen, prepared, ½ cup	0.28		
Shrimp, cooked, 3 ounces*		0.12	0.12
Refried beans, canned, vegetarian, ½ cup	0.21		
Lobster, cooked, 3 ounces*	0.04	0.07	0.1
Tuna, light, canned in water, drained, 3 ounces*		0.17	0.02
Tilapia, cooked, 3 ounces*	0.04	0.11	
Scallops, cooked, 3 ounces*		0.09	0.06
Cod, Pacific, cooked, 3 ounces*		0.1	0.04
Tuna, yellowfin, cooked 3 ounces*		0.09	0.01
Kidney beans, canned ½ cup	0.1		
Baked beans, canned, vegetarian, ½ cup	0.07		
Ground beef, 85% lean, cooked, 3 ounces**	0.04		
Bread, whole wheat, 1 slice	0.04		
Egg, cooked, 1 egg		0.03	
Chicken, breast, roasted, 3 ounces		0.02	0.01
Milk, low-fat (1%), 1 cup	0.01		

*Except as noted, the USDA database does not specify whether fish are farmed or wild caught.

**The USDA database does not specify whether beef is grass fed or grain fed.

Source: https://ods.od.nih.gov/factsheets/Omega3FattyAcids-HealthProfessional

fish at least 2-3 times during your PMSC Week, or taking a 1,000 mg fish oil supplement daily. You should be avoiding red meat anyway, so why not replace hormone-imbalancing red meats with fatty fish full of the omega-3s that you need?

For vegetarians and vegans, I recommend adding a spoonful of flax or chia seeds to your meals, or taking 1,000 mg of algae oil supplements daily.

FOCUS ON ALA OMEGA-3S

Regardless of your dietary needs, remember that you should focus on increasing your intake of ALA omega-3s. These are only found in plant-based sources, and are listed under "Seeds" and "Plant Oils" above. I think the easiest ones to find in America are flaxseed, chia seeds, walnuts, flaxseed oil, and canola oil. For best results, I strongly recommend adding food sources of ALA omega-3s to your diets.

Plant-based sources of omega-3s should be consumed raw, and an easy way to add them to your diet is to sprinkle a spoonful of the seeds on your food – in smoothies, on top of salads, in oatmeal, on top of avocado toast. The possibilities are truly only limited by your preference and Pinterest boards. My go-to method is making fruit smoothies and adding flax and chia seeds – your tastebuds won't even notice them, but your uterus sure will!

For meal recommendations that are high in omega-3s and also avoid the hormone-imbalancing foods listed in Chapter 3, please see Appendix III.

ADDITIONAL BENEFITS OF OMEGA-3 FATTY ACIDS

The focus of this book is to prevent PMS, but I want to continue to stress that all of the methods that prevent PMS will also benefit and improve your overall health and lifestyle. Omega-3 fatty acids are not only great for balancing hormones, but they have also been proven to have these additional health benefits:

- <u>Menstrual benefits:</u> Studies prove that dietary supplementation with omega-3 fatty acids is more effective in treating dysmenorrhea (painful menstrual cycles) than ibuprofen.

- <u>Cosmetic benefits:</u> Omega-3 fatty acids can improve your skin and hair – they reduce the risk of acne and premature aging, and also help protect your skin from the effects of sun damage.

- <u>Mental benefits:</u> Regularly consuming omega-3s fights anxiety and depression, and has been proven by epidemiological and experimental studies to be equally as effective as prescription anti-depressant medication in the prevention or treatment of depressive disorders.

- <u>General health benefits:</u>

  - Omega-3s are anti-inflammatory, and studies show that consistently consuming omega-3s leads to long-term reduced inflammation.

  - Omega-3 fatty acids can improve insulin resistance, and reduce inflammation and heart disease risk factors in people with metabolic syndrome.

  - Regularly consuming omega-3s improves heart health and decreases your risk for heart disease

- and stroke.
- Eating omega-3 fatty acids is linked to a reduced risk of macular degeneration, one of the world's leading causes of permanent eye damage and blindness.
- Omega-3 fatty acids can help fight several autoimmune diseases, including type 1 diabetes, rheumatoid arthritis, ulcerative colitis, and Crohn's disease.
- Omega-3 consumption is linked to reduced cancer risk in both men and women.
- Omega-3s have been shown to increase calcium absorption, retention, and deposition in bone, and to improve bone strength and health.

Bottom line: omega-3s — one of our *essential* fatty acids — do wonders for women! From head to toe, omega-3s contribute to every single cell in our bodies. Eat them!

IS THERE ANYTHING ELSE I SHOULD EAT TO AVOID PMS?

Why yes, there is! Eat fresh fruits and vegetables. I think we all know that fruits and vegetables are good for you, but did you know that they also support balanced hormones? Fresh fruits and vegetables all have anti-inflammatory and antioxidant properties which help to balance hormones. You should get at least 5 servings of fruits and vegetables daily. Dark leafy greens (collards, turnip greens, kale, spinach, callaloo, etc) are some of the best sources of hormone-balancing vegetables. You can reap the benefits of fresh fruits and vegetables whether they are eaten raw, cooked, juiced, or blended into smoothies.

CONCLUSION: DIETARY CHANGES FOR HORMONAL BALANCE

Successfully cutting out the hormone-imbalancing foods and adding hormone-balancing foods during your Pre-Menstrual Self-Care Week _will_ have a positive affect on your PMS symptoms. In addition, many doctors have successfully completed studies proving that permanently cutting out, or seriously reducing, your intake of the hormone-imbalancing foods will have a significant positive effect on various medical problems and your overall health. This book is about avoiding PMS, but, I recommend that you consider changing your dietary habits for good. Food is meant to nourish our bodies and our minds, and there's no reason to consume food that is detrimental to either.

CHAPTER 5

Exercising for Hormonal Balance

When I first began to solve my PMS problems, exercising was the hardest thing for me to change. I've never liked exercising. I've never had any health problems or weight problems, and since I've always felt great about my body image, I never felt the need to exercise. Frankly, I was pretty lazy! When my PMS symptoms got out of control though, I decided that I'd rather exercise than have my skin breakout every month, or suffer from painful breasts. So I made the change and committed to exercising during my

Pre-Menstrual Self-Care Week. My skin and my uterus are glad that I did!

HOW DOES EXERCISING AFFECT HORMONES?

We all know that exercising is good for your health, but how is it related to PMS? Studies have proven that exercising releases dopamine, which decreases stress, and releases serotonin, which boosts your mood and promotes good sleeping (we'll talk more about using sleep and stress management to avoid PMS in Chapter 6). In addition, exercising also affects your body's production of estrogen.

During your Pre-Menstrual Self-Care Week, when your estrogen levels are naturally changing due to the luteal phase, it is imperative that you exercise to manage production of estrogen and serotonin. In particular, doing cardio will help to balance your hormones. Cardio, short for cardiovascular exercise, is any movement that increases your heart rate and blood circulation throughout the body. This includes activities like walking, biking, running, aerobics, dancing, swimming, and spin classes. During your PMSC Week, you should do at least 30 minutes of cardio daily in order to balance your body's production of estrogen and serotonin.

ADDING CARDIO TO YOUR PMS PREVENTION PLAN

If you already have a workout routine, that's awesome! Just make sure to get your heart pumping for at least 30 minutes every day during your PMSC Week. This might mean adding more cardio to your current routine, or doing shorter and more intense workouts during your PMSC Week.

If you've been wanting to get more active, but haven't gotten around to it, now is the perfect time to start! Living a PMS-free life is great motivation. I'm a big fan of getting the most out of everything I do, so I always recommend women choose an activity that provides more than one benefit. For example, exercising to balance your hormones is a great reason to join a gym or an outdoor club, or to learn a new sport. This way, not only are you balancing your hormones and getting healthier, but you're also learning something new, or meeting new people. Pick something that makes you feel GOOD about yourself. Go outdoors if you like being in nature, or join an adults intramural team if you're competitive (or a children's team if you hate losing). Take an African dance class to learn something new, or a pole dancing class to feel sexy!

Don't want to spend any money? There are literally millions of free apps and YouTube videos for at-home cardio workouts. There is no special clothing or equipment required to do cardio in the comfort of your own home. This means that money is NOT an excuse to avoid working out during your PMSC Week!

Can't find the time? Remember, our PMSC Week is a week of supreme self-care. So you should do your best to only schedule activities that improve your physical, emotional, and mental health. Take a good look at your schedule. Any life coach, or your mom, can tell you that we make time for the things that we want to do. The Nielsen Company reports that the average American spends nearly one hour per day on social media, and nearly six hours per day watching videos or TV. These are activities that will not help alleviate your PMS symptoms. Do yourself a favor and schedule some time for cardio! It's just for one week out of the month, so don't let time be an excuse not to workout.

Some of you might truly have extremely busy lifestyles. Maybe you're a high-powered executive or work long hours at multiple jobs. If you've looked at your schedule, and you truly cannot make time for a 30-minute workout, then I recommend that you get in as much cardio as possible whenever you can throughout the day. Take the stairs instead of the elevator. Deliberately pick a parking spot that's further away from your destination. Walk one bus or train station further away from your usual stop. Perhaps you can commit to doing 10 minutes of cardio a day instead of 30. Be creative! If it gets your heart rate up, then it counts as cardio (wink wink). If you're currently not exercising at all, then incorporating even these small changes will affect your hormone levels and have a positive effect on your PMS symptoms.

EXERCISING FOR SELF-CARE

Remember that one of the reasons we track our period is to be able to properly schedule our lives so that we can prepare for and maximize our Pre-Menstrual Self-Care Week. If you want to see results, then you need to be committed to balancing your hormones. Changing your life to make time for cardio exercises is a worthwhile change to make! Doing cardio exercises not only improves PMS symptoms, but is also great for weight loss, heart health, muscle strength and maintenance, increasing metabolism, lowering blood pressure, regulating blood sugar, and improving brain function. This is why I believe it's good to view your pre-menstrual week as a week of self-care and not sacrifice: all of the things that you should do to avoid PMS are things that will also improve your physical, mental, and emotional health.

CHAPTER 6

Lifestyle Changes for Hormonal Balance

Most of us do not live in such a way to maximize our physical, mental, and spiritual health. We're not getting enough sleep; our stress levels are higher than ever; anxiety and mental illness are on the rise; and many people of all ages complain that they are unable to make real connections with people or spend quality time with their loved ones. This is especially true for women, because our lifestyles can contribute to unbalanced hormones. This chapter is about balancing your hormones during your Pre-Menstrual Self-

Care Week using sleep management, stress management, and relaxation and mood management.

SLEEP MANAGEMENT

Getting enough sleep is essential to living a healthy lifestyle. Epidemiologic and laboratory studies in adults indicate that sleep deprivation results in metabolic and endocrine alternations, as well as increased hunger and appetite. Sleep deprivation also has negative effects on your mood, your brain, and your overall health. In fact, people who don't get enough sleep are more likely to get cardiovascular disease, diabetes, and high blood pressure.

But did you know that lack of sleep can affect hormone production and cause an imbalance in your hormones during your PMSC Week? Research shows that hormone fluctuations during a woman's menstrual cycle (and menopause) can affect sleep patterns. In turn, sleep deprivation can affect hormone levels in a sleepless vicious cycle. Remember from Chapter 1 that one of the symptoms of PMS is fatigue – by not getting enough sleep, you'll not only be tired from lack of sleep, but you will also throw your hormones out of whack and cause even more fatigue! The cycle is so vicious. That's why it's important to get enough sleep during your PMSC Week so that you can balance your hormones and avoid a sleepless vicious cycle.

What is "enough" sleep? Doctors recommend 7-9 hours of sleep every night, but only you can determine how much sleep is right for you. Balancing your hormones will require you to get to know yourself and your body. In my normal life, I get about 6-8 hours of sleep every night, but during my Pre-Menstrual Self-Care Week, I make time for at least 8-10 hours of sleep every day. During your PMSC Week, make sure to plan time to get at least 8 hours of sleep every night. No staying up late watching Netflix or reading. No late nights out with the girls. No cramming for tests til dark-thirty in the morning. If you have children, put them to bed early.

For me, 10 hours of sleep is ideal. When I sleep for 10 hours, I feel rested and refreshed. When I wake up after 10 hours of sleep, I don't feel the need to drink coffee, which we've learned should be avoided during the PMSC Week.

For many of you, getting more sleep during your Pre-Menstrual Self-Care Week will also help you to avoid drinking caffeine.

How you sleep is just as important as the amount of time you sleep. For some of you, using your PMSC Week as a reason to get more sleep is great news! If you're a nocturnal creature like me; however, this may be a bit difficult for you. I have found that I'm most productive at night, and I've always had difficulty when trying to fall asleep at a normal time. Here are some suggestions from medical experts to help you avoid insomnia, fall asleep, and sleep better:

- Create and stick to a regular and consistent sleeping schedule. Maintain a strict time to go to bed and wake up to develop a routine.
- Avoid taking naps during the day because naps make you less sleepy at night.
- Try not to exercise three hours before the time you go to sleep. Regular exercising in the day, however, is beneficial for sleep.
- Avoid alcohol and caffeine within 8 hours of bedtime.

- Avoid snacking and eating late at night, which will affect your quality of sleep.
- Follow a bedtime routine like brushing your teeth, washing face, prayer for 2 minutes. These cues send psychological signals to alert your mind and body that it's time to sleep.
- Limit the use of electronic appliances (television, laptop, & cell phone) 1 hour before bed. These devices emit light and disrupt your body's biological clock.
- Meditate to improve your focus, mindfulness, relieve stress and reduce anxiety.
- Establish an evening routing.
- Take over-the-counter or prescription sleep medication.

As we've seen in previous chapters, during your PMSC Week you should exercise and avoid caffeine, which should help you sleep. What helped me even further was to establish an evening and a morning routine.

This is my evening routine that helps me fall asleep, and

my morning routine that helps me wake up and begin my day in a way that is best for me:

Evening routine: *1 hour before intended sleep time*

- Take a shower and prepare for bed
- Listen to relaxing instrumental music
- Do 10-15 minutes of yoga
- Refrain from eating or drinking
- Refrain from any brain-stimulating activities such as reading
- Refrain from using any electronic devices
- Take 5-10 minutes to write affirmations, write things I'm grateful for, and write to congratulate myself on completing a successful day
- Take 5-10 minutes to do a brain dump (a technique to declutter your mind and thoughts)

Morning routine: *1 hour before any work begins*

- Drink 1 cup of water mixed with apple cider vinegar or lemon juice
- Take a shower

- Listen to upbeat music

- Do 10-15 minutes of yoga

- Get dressed

- Avoid any human interaction

- Refrain from using any electronic devices

- Take 5-10 minutes to write affirmations, write things
    I'm grateful for, and write about my excitement for
    the upcoming great day

- Review the day's to-do list and visualize the day

These routines work very well for me. It's extremely important to sleep and sleep well during your PMSC Week, and developing a routine can help you to do so.

When I've had a really good night's sleep, it's easier for me to wake up and begin my day, which cuts down on stress – instead of hitting the snooze button ten times, then running around frantically in the morning, I can easily wake up an hour before I need to be productive, and take the time to go through my routine to best prepare for my day.

This leads us right into the next lifestyle change to balance your hormones: avoiding stress.

STRESS MANAGEMENT

Stress is another vicious cycle – hormone fluctuations can affect stress, and stress can affect hormone production. Therefore, it's extremely important to remain stress-free during your PMSC Week in order to help balance your hormones.

Cortisol is a steroid hormone. In response to stress, extra cortisol is released to help the body respond appropriately. High cortisol levels lower estrogen levels. When estrogen is lowered from unrelenting stress and cortisol production, female hormone imbalance symptoms such as hot flashes, night sweats, sleep problems, and mood swings can be exacerbated. High levels of cortisol have also been proven to negatively affect menstruation. These effects could mean short cycles (less than 28 days), long cycles (more than 28 days), dysmenorrhea (painful menstruation), oligomenorrhea (infrequent or irregular menstruation), or could even be as severe as amenorrhoea (no menstruation at all).

Basically, women should be pampered like queens for

our entire lives and only spend our time doing whatever it is that brings us joy. Until that day comes though, you must manage and reduce your stress. Remember, YOU are scheduling this week! Schedule it to completely avoid, or at least minimize, experiences and interactions that cause you stress. If you can avoid working overtime, do it. If you can dodge that nagging relative for a week, do it. Do as much meal prep as possible to cut down on your work load. Schedule your visit to the DMV before or after your PMSC Week. Even small stress reductions will have a big impact on your hormonal balance, and the overall quality of your life.

External stress, can only be controlled so much. After all, it's unlikely that you'll quit your job or close your business to prevent PMS! We have complete control over internal stress, or emotional stress, but this is often much harder to target. This kind of stress can be caused by pressure you put on yourself, feelings of insecurity, or trauma.

Stress can only be changed and properly managed if you're willing to make a change. Balancing your hormones through the methods detailed so far in this book will help you avoid stress. Here are some additional stress management tips:

- Address emotional issues. Seek professional assistance if you need it.
- Avoid toxic people
- Spend time in nature
- Do breathing exercises
- If you smoke, stop.

There are numerous books, articles, and blogs written to help women lower stress. If you live a high-stress lifestyle, please take the time to seek out and consult these resources.

RELAXATION AND MOOD MANAGEMENT

If you successfully remove foods from your diet that unbalance your hormones, add omega-3 fatty acids to your diet, and do cardio exercise during your PMSC Week, then you shouldn't suffer from mood swings at all. However, you should still pay special attention to your mood, especially if you live a high-stress life or if your PMS symptoms usually include mood swings or feelings of depression. If you plan your week right, you can spend an entire seven days stress-free and in a great mood! Schedule as much time as possible for relaxing activities and activities that make you feel good. This could be as extravagant as a spa getaway vacation once a month, or as simple as lighting a nice candle.

Do not underestimate the power of your five senses to affect your mood. Listen to music that is relaxing or soothing, or music that is happy and makes you feel great. Watch stand-up comedy or listen to comedy podcasts to get some laughs and keep your mood up. Use aromatherapy to make you feel happy or relaxed. Use your favorite bath and body products to feel great about yourself. If you find taking long baths to be relaxing, schedule time to take a few baths during your Pre-Menstrual Self-Care Week. If you find yoga or meditation relaxing, then schedule time for those activities.

Whatever works for you, DO IT! Make time every

single day during your Pre-Menstrual Self-Care Week to laugh, to relax, and to feel great about yourself.

CHAPTER 7

Putting It All Together

How can you take all of this information and put it to use? It will definitely take some effort, but it's easier than it may seem!

Remember the goal: to balance your hormones through diet, exercise, and living well. Again, you may see some reduction in symptoms if you make some of the changes, but you will *definitely* be free from PMS, in as soon as one menstrual cycle, if you make <u>all</u> of the changes. For best results, I recommend that you plan as much of your Pre-

Menstrual Self-Care Week as your life allows. This is another reason to track your menstrual cycle – to be able to make the appropriate schedule. If you had an important presentation to give on a Wednesday, you wouldn't *deliberately* make yourself feel awful that entire week, would you? Take that same mindset with your menstrual cycle – instead of deliberately making it hard for yourself, do your best to set yourself up for success. Plan your meals, plan your work, plan your exercise, plan your relaxation time, plan your errands.

I have created an example one-day schedule in a Pre-Menstrual Self-Care Week to give you an idea of how you can take all of the information provided in this book and put it together:

7am – 8am: Wake up feeling refreshed. Do a morning routine and get ready for work.
Breakfast - fruit smoothie with chia and flax seeds, or oatmeal with chia and flax seeds.
Drink peppermint tea which is naturally invigorating.

8am – 9am: Commute to work. Listen to happy music or a comedy podcast to keep your mood up.

9am – 5pm: Work. If your job permits it, listen to happy music while at work.

Lunch - Salmon salad with a dairy-free dressing. Drink plenty of water.

Try not to spend the whole day sitting. Take some time to walk around the office, or step outside for a few minutes.

5pm – 6pm: Commute back home. Listen to happy music or a comedy podcast to keep your mood up.

6pm – 6:30pm: Do some cardio exercises.

6:30pm – 7:30pm: Prepare a simple Mexican food dinner – Chipotle chicken or tofu, Mexican rice, cumin black beans, and avocado slices.

Put the leftovers in a tupperware for lunch the next day.

Prepare tomorrow's breakfast – prep overnight oats or prep frozen fruits and seeds for a smoothie.

7:30pm: Do something fun and/or relaxing! Watch a movie (nothing sad!), read a book, do some journaling, catch up on that in-progress knitting project, do a fun art project with your kids, take a long bubble bath, enjoy some chamomile tea.

9pm: Begin sleep routine and prepare to fall sleep.

10pm: Get extra sleep!

This example day incorporates all of the hormone-balancing methods that have been discussed in this book:

<u>Diet</u> – In this example, the woman has completely avoided hormone-imbalancing foods and has consumed a sufficient amount of omega-3s.

<u>Exercise</u> – In this example, the woman has completed a sufficient amount of cardio exercise.

<u>Lifestyle</u> – In this example, the woman has minimized stress and maximized sleep and relaxation.

These days, few people are working 9-to-5s, but this example schedule can give you an idea about how to structure your days during your PMSC Week. It can be modified to suit your work schedule or your lifestyle, and of course you can create your own schedule.

When making your schedule, set yourself up for success by avoiding places where hormone-imbalancing foods or activities will be present. If you are a salaried employee, avoid stress by sticking to your required eight hours of work per day and avoiding overtime during your PMSC Week. If you are an hourly worker, try to schedule your shifts in such a way that allows you to get the best sleep. If you're a business owner or a stay-at-home mom, try to schedule yourself for a week that prioritizes getting good sleep and minimizing stress. Whenever possible, avoid attending social events where only hormone-imbalancing foods will be served, like happy hours at bars or Krispy Kreme grand openings.

Remember, your period is not a hindrance! This is a week of supreme self-care and self-improvement. Go to bed early, get a lot of sleep, and wake up fresh. Live a stress-free life, listen to music that keeps you in a good mood, and exercise. Eat good food that will nourish your mind, body, and soul. Relax, take good care of yourself, and love yourself!

Living a Great Life as a Woman

Successfully balancing your hormones through diet, exercise, and the lifestyle changes mentioned in this book is the solution to PMS prevention. If you follow the full regimen described in this book, then you will see results as soon as your next menstrual cycle. Your hormones will remain in balance, and your body will immediately respond to the positive changes so that you can start living PMS-free immediately. Following these methods each month will not only prevent PMS, but will also improve your overall quality of life. You'll have better periods, be amazingly healthy, AND feel great!

After a few months of following the Pre-Menstrual Self-Care Week method, I realized that my period wasn't ruining my life at all, but that my life had been ruining my period. By changing my lifestyle in order to ease my PMS, I discovered that I actually lived a better life. Each month I enjoyed a week of self-care, no stress, and relaxation. When my period began at the end of that week, I rewarded myself throughout my menstruation with cake and wine! It felt so good to not only gain back two weeks of my life every month, but to transform those two weeks into a week dedicated to self-care and a week dedicated to treating myself.

I encourage you to do the same – plan your Pre-Menstrual Self-Care Week, then treat yourself to nice things during your menstruation. You may not be able to change the whole world's view of women and menstruation, but you can change your own view and your own life. You're not sick or flawed, and your menstrual cycle is not a plight or a burden. I hope that if you've made it this far, that you decide to love yourself as a woman and to live a better life in your womanhood.

Thanks for reading, and good luck ladies!

Appendices

Meat-based sources of omega-3 fatty acids

- Salmon

- Mackerel

- Tuna

- Herring

- Sardines

- Oysters

- Mussels

- Omega-3 fortified eggs

- Omega-3 fortified yogurt

- Omega-3 fortified milk and milk beverages

Plant-based sources of omega-3 fatty acids

- Algae, algal oil

- Flaxseed, flaxseed oil

- Perilla (also called shiso or kkaennip) seeds, perilla
  seed oil

- Lingonberry seeds, lingonberry seed oil

- Hemp seeds, hemp oil

- Camelina seeds, camelina seed oil

- Chia seeds

- Walnuts

- Kiwifruit seeds

- Pumpkin seeds

- Sea buckthorn

- Wheat germ oil

- Soybean oil

- Canola (also called rapeseed) oil

- Omega-3 fortified juices

- Omega-3 fortified soy beverages

PMS Prevention Meal Plan Ideas

Breakfast

- Fruit smoothies or smoothie bowls with chia and flax seeds

- Bowl of fresh fruit sprinkled with chia and flax seeds

- Oatmeal with banana and chia and flax seeds

- Sugar-free granola cereal with almond milk (or any non-dairy plant-based milk)

- Tofu scramble with toast and honey

- Avocado toast with flax seeds

- Egg-free breakfast burrito

Lunch

- Chicken, turkey, or veggie sub sandwich (no mayo)
- Salmon, chicken, or garden salad with walnuts and a
  dairy-free dressing (add flaxseeds or flax oil for
  more omega-3s)

Meat-based Dinners

- Cajun salmon with wild rice and broccoli
- Harissa stewed chicken and rice
- Chicken tikka masala
- Garlic and herb baked fish (no salt) with brussel
  sprouts, spinach, and quinoa
- Mexican bowl with chicken, mexican rice, and black
  beans
- Jamaican jerk chicken with callaloo, plantain, and rice
  and peas
- Red beans with rice and green beans (no pork, beef,
  or other red meat)
- Chicken pasta with tomato basil sauce
- BBQ chicken, corn on the cob, and collard greens
- Chicken pad thai (no egg)

Vegetarian/Vegan Dinners

- BBQ tofu, corn on the cob, honey roasted sweet
  potatoes, and collard greens
- Chickpea curry
- Mexican bowl with tofu sofritas, mexican rice, and
  black beans
- Vegetarian lentil soup
- Black-eyed peas, West African jollof rice, and yams
- Caribbean rice and peas with plantain and callaloo
- Vegetable pasta
- Tofu pad thai (no egg)

Beverages

- Drink water (or sparkling water)
- Fruit-infused water
- No-sugar-added organic fruit and vegetable juices
- Sugar-free kombucha
- Golden milk
- Caffeine-free teas (peppermint tea, hibiscus tea,
  chamomile tea, etc)

REFERENCES

Chapter 1

1. Arora, Sarika. "PMS Symptoms." *Women's Health Network.* https://www.womenshealthnetwork.com/pms-and-menstruation/pms-symptoms.aspx.
2. Cabeca, Anna. *The Hormone Fix.* Ballantine Books, 1 edition, 2019, February 26.
3. Northrup, Christiane. *The Wisdom of Menopause.* Bantam Books, 2001.
4. Miller-Keane Encyclopedia and Dictionary of Medicine, Nursing, and Allied Health, Seventh Edition. Copyright 2003 by Saunders, an imprint of Elsevier, Inc.
5. Greenwood, Beth. "How Does Caffeine Affect Estrogen Levels?" *Livestrong.com.* https://www.livestrong.com/article/503844-how-does-caffeine-affect-estrogen-levels/.
6. Fletcher, Jenna. "What are the phases of the menstrual cycle?" *Medical News Today.* https://www.medicalnewstoday.com/articles/326906.
7. Watson, Stephanie. "Stages of the Menstrual Cycle." *Healthline.* https://www.healthline.com/health/womens-health/stages-of-menstrual-cycle.
8. Hawkins, Shannon M. and Matzuk, Martin M. "Menstrual Cycle: Basic Biology." *The New York Academy of Sciences,* Volume 1135, Issue 1. 2008, July 25. https://nyaspubs.onlinelibrary.wiley.com/doi/abs/10.1196/annals.1429.018.

Chapter 2

1. Johnson, Traci C. "What Is a Normal Period? *WebMD.* https://www.webmd.com/women/normal-period.
2. Johns Hopkins Medicine: "Menstrual Cycle: An Overview."
3. Cleveland Clinic: "Menstrual Cycle."

4. Womenshealth.gov: "Menstruation and the menstrual cycle."

5. Covey, Stephen R. *The 7 Habits of Highly Effective People.* 1989, Free Press.

Chapter 3

1. Northrup, Christiane. *The Wisdom of Menopause.* Bantam Books, 2001.

2. Gunnars, Kris. "Coconut Sugar – A Healthy Sugar Alternative or a Big, Fat Lie?" *Healthline.* https://www.healthline.com/nutrition/coconut-sugar.

3. Deville, Lauren. "How Caffeine Affects Your Hormones." https://www.drlaurendeville.com/articles/caffeine-affects-hormones/.

4. Walsh, Bryan. "Coffee and hormones: Here's how coffee really affects your health: *Precision Nutrition.* https://www.precisionnutrition.com/coffee-and-hormones.

5. Wszelaki, Magdalena. "11 Ways Coffee Impacts Your Hormones and How to Substitute It." *Hormones & Balance.* https://hormonesbalance.com/articles/11-ways-coffee-impacts-your-hormones-and-how-to-substitute-it/.

6. Lam, Michael. "The Role of Adrenal Fatigue in Estrogen Hormone Dominance." *DrLam Coaching.* https://www.drlamcoaching.com/adrenal-fatigue/symptoms/estrogen-hormone-dominance/.

7. Moody, Liz. "These 8 Foods Are Wreaking Havoc On Your Hormones." *mindbodygreen.* https://www.mindbodygreen.com/0-29200/these-8-foods-are-wreaking-havoc-on-your-hormones.html.

8. Maita, Lorraine. "Foods that Affect Hormone Levels and Health." *HowToLiveYounger.com.* https://howtoliveyounger.com/foods-affect-hormone-levels-health/.

9. "Complex carbohydrates." *MedlinePlus.* https://medlineplus.gov/ency/imagepages/19529.htm.

10. Benninghoven, Danica. "What Are Refined Sugars?" *Livestrong.com.* https://www.livestrong.com/article/67126-refined-sugars/.

11. Gearing, Mary E. "Natural and Added Sugars: Two Sides of the Same Coin." *Science in the News.* 2015, October 5. http://sitn.hms.harvard.edu/flash/2015/natural-and-added-sugars-two-sides-of-the-same-coin/.

12. Bauer, Joy. "How Food Affects PMS." *JoyBauer.com.*

http://joybauer.com/pms/how-food-affects-pms/.

13. "What to eat and what to avoid for menstrual cramps." *LiverDoctor*. https://www.liverdoctor.com/what-to-eat-and-what-to-avoid-for-menstrual-cramps/.

14. Ciccotelli, Valentina. "Sodium Balance and Menstrual Cycle." *Università degli Studi di Torino*. 2012, May 25. http://flipper.diff.org/apptagsaccount/items/4474.

15. White, Krishna Wood. "PMS, Cramps, and Irregular Periods." *Nemours*. https://kidshealth.org/en/teens/menstrual-problems.html.

16. Anniga, Jan. "Side Effects of Ingesting Too Much Salt." *SFGATE*. https://healthyeating.sfgate.com/side-effects-ingesting-much-salt-6242.html.

17. "Eating processed food." https://www.nhs.uk/live-well/eat-well/what-are-processed-foods/.

18. "Processed Food: What Is the Purpose of Food Processing?" https://www.eufic.org/en/food-production/article/processed-food-qa.

19. Smith, Amy. "How do processed foods affect your health?" *Medical News Today*. https://www.medicalnewstoday.com/articles/318630.

20. Collins, Sonya. "Hidden Dangers of Ultraprocessed Foods." *WebMD*. https://www.webmd.com/diet/news/20200221/hidden-dangers-of-ultraprocessed-foods.

21. Fuhrman, Joel. "The Hidden Dangers of Fast and Processed Food." *National Center for Biotechnology Information, U.S. National Library of Medicine*. 2018, April 3. https://www.ncbi.nlm.nih.gov/pmc/articles/PMC6146358/.

Chapter 4

1. Merle, Benedicte MJ, Benlian, Pascale, Puche, Nathalie, Bassols, Ana, Delcourt, Ceclie, Souied, Eric H., and Nutrional AMD Treatment 2 Study Group. "Circulating omega-3 Fatty Acids and Neovascular Age-Related Macular Degeneration." *National Center for Biotechnology Information, U.S. National Library of Medicine*. 2014, March 28. https://www.ncbi.nlm.nih.gov/pubmed/24557349.

2. McCusker, Meagen M. and Grant-Kels, Jane M. "Healing fats 2. of the skin: the structural and immunologic roles of the ω-6 and ω-3 fatty acids." *Clinics in Dermatology*. Volume 28, Issue 4, July–August 2010, Pages 440-451. https://www.sciencedirect.com/science/article/abs/pii/S073808

1X10000441.

3. Brusch, Charles A. and Johnson, Edward T. "A New Dietary Regimen for Arthritis. Value of Cod Liver Oil on a Fasting Stomach." *J Natl Med Assoc.* 1959 Jul; 51(4): 266-270, 295. https://www.ncbi.nlm.nih.gov/pmc/articles/PMC2641566/?page=2.

4. Ladesich JB, Pottala JV, Romaker A, Harris WS. Membrane level of omega-3 docosahexaenoic acid is associated with severity of obstructive sleep apnea. *J Clin Sleep Med.* 2011;7(4):391-396. doi:10.5664/JCSM.1198. https://www.ncbi.nlm.nih.gov/pubmed/21897776.

5. Zafari, Mandana, Behmanesh, Fereshteh, and Mohammadi, Azar A. "Comparison of the effect of fish oil and ibuprofen on treatment of severe pain in primary dysmenorrhea." *Caspian J Intern Med.* 2011 Summer; 2(3): 279–282. https://www.ncbi.nlm.nih.gov/pmc/articles/PMC3770499/.

6. Harel Z, Biro FM, Kottenhahn RK, Rosenthal SL. Supplementation with omega-3 polyunsaturated fatty acids in the management of dysmenorrhea in adolescents. *Am J Obstet Gynecol.* 1996;174(4):1335-1338. doi:10.1016/s0002-9378(96)70681-6. https://www.ncbi.nlm.nih.gov/pubmed/8623866.

7. Kruger MC, Horrobin DF. Calcium metabolism, osteoporosis and essential fatty acids: a review. *Prog Lipid Res.* 1997;36(2-3):131-151. doi:10.1016/s0163-7827(97)00007-6. https://www.ncbi.nlm.nih.gov/pubmed/9624425.

8. Li, Jingjing, Xun, Pengcheng, Zamora, Daisy, Sood, Akshay, Liu, Kiang, Daviglus, Martha, Iribarren, Carlos, Jacobs Jr., David, Shikany, James M. and He, Ka. "Intakes of long-chain omega-3 (n-3) PUFAs and fish in relation to incidence of asthma among American young adults: the CARDIA study." *Am J Clin Nutr.* 2013 Jan; 97(1): 181–186. Published online 2012 Nov 28. doi: 10.3945/ajcn.112.041145. https://www.ncbi.nlm.nih.gov/pmc/articles/PMC3522136/.

9. Laerum BN, Wentzel-Larsen T, Gulsvik A, et al. Relationship of fish and cod oil intake with adult asthma. *Clin Exp Allergy.* 2007;37(11):1616-1623. doi:10.1111/j.1365-2222.2007.02821.x. https://www.ncbi.nlm.nih.gov/pubmed/17877766/.

10. Yang, Huan, Xun, Pengcheng, and He, Ka. "Fish and Fish Oil Intake in Relation to Risk of Asthma: A Systematic Review and Meta-Analysis." *PLoS One.* 2013; 8(11): e80048. Published online 2013 Nov 12. doi: 10.1371/journal.pone.0080048. https://www.ncbi.nlm.nih.gov/pmc/articles/PMC3827145/.

11. "Omega-3 Fatty Acids. Fact Sheet for Health Professionals."
    National Institutes of Heath.
    https://ods.od.nih.gov/factsheets/Omega3FattyAcids-HealthProf
    essional/.

12. "Fish Oil (EPA & DHA)." *Nutrition Express.*
    https://www.nutritionexpress.com/supplements/omega+3-6-9+fa
    tty+acids/fish+oil.

13. Terry PD, Terry JB, Rohan TE. Long-chain (n-3) fatty acid
    intake and risk of cancers of the breast and the prostate: recent
    epidemiological studies, biological mechanisms, and directions
    for future research. *J Nutr.* 2004;134(12 Suppl):3412S-3420S.
    doi:10.1093/jn/134.12.3412S,
    https://www.ncbi.nlm.nih.gov/pubmed/15570047/.

14. Theodoratou E, McNeill G, Cetnarskyj R, et al. Dietary fatty
    acids and colorectal cancer: a case-control study. *Am J Epidemiol.*
    2007;166(2):181-195. doi:10.1093/aje/kwm063.
    https://www.ncbi.nlm.nih.gov/pubmed/17493949.

15. Benton D. The impact of diet on anti-social, violent and
    criminal behaviour. *Neurosci Biobehav Rev.* 2007;31(5):752-774.
    doi:10.1016/j.neubiorev.2007.02.002.
    https://www.ncbi.nlm.nih.gov/pubmed/17433442.

16. Peet M, Stokes C. Omega-3 fatty acids in the treatment of
    psychiatric disorders. *Drugs.* 2005;65(8):1051-1059.
    doi:10.2165/00003495-200565080-00002.
    https://www.ncbi.nlm.nih.gov/pubmed/15907142.

17. Grosso, Giuseppe, Galvano, Fabio, Marventano, Stefano,
    Malaguarnera, Michele, Bucolo, Claudio, Drago, Filippo, and
    Caraci, Filippo. "Omega-3 Fatty Acids and Depression: Scientific
    Evidence and Biological Mechanisms." *Oxid Med Cell Longev.*
    2014; 2014: 313570. Published online 2014 Mar 18. doi:
    10.1155/2014/313570.
    https://www.ncbi.nlm.nih.gov/pmc/articles/PMC3976923/.

18. Berbert AA, Kondo CR, Almendra CL, Matsuo T, Dichi I.
    Supplementation of fish oil and olive oil in patients with
    rheumatoid arthritis. *Nutrition.* 2005;21(2):131-136.
    doi:10.1016/j.nut.2004.03.023.
    https://www.ncbi.nlm.nih.gov/pubmed/15723739.

19. Papadia C, Coruzzi A, Montana C, Di Mario F, Franzè A, Forbes
    A. Omega-3 fatty acids in the maintenance of ulcerative colitis.
    JRSM Short Rep. 2010;1(1):15. Published 2010 Jun 30.
    doi:10.1258/shorts.2010.010004.
    https://www.ncbi.nlm.nih.gov/pubmed/21103107.

20. Lofvengor, JE, Andersoon, T., Carlsson, P-O, Dorkhan, M., Groop, L., Martinelli, M., Tuomi, T., Wolk, A., and Carlsson, S. "Fatty fish consumption and risk of latent autoimmune diabetes in adults." *Nutr Diabetes.* 2014 Oct; 4(10): e139. Published online 2014 Oct 20. doi: 10.1038/nutd.2014.36. https://www.ncbi.nlm.nih.gov/pmc/articles/PMC4216999/.

21. Spencer Elsa H., Ferdowslan, Hope R., Barnard, Neal D. "Diet and acne: a review of the evidence." *International Journal of Dermatology.* Volume 48, Issue 4. https://onlinelibrary.wiley.com/doi/full/10.1111/j.1365-4632.2009.04002.x.

22. Calder PC. n-3 polyunsaturated fatty acids, inflammation, and inflammatory diseases. *Am J Clin Nutr.* 2006;83(6 Suppl):1505S-1519S. doi:10.1093/ajcn/83.6.1505S. https://www.ncbi.nlm.nih.gov/pubmed/16841861.

23. Simopoulos AP. Omega-3 fatty acids in inflammation and autoimmune diseases. *J Am Coll Nutr.* 2002;21(6):495-505. doi:10.1080/07315724.2002.10719248. https://www.ncbi.nlm.nih.gov/pubmed/12480795.

24. Robinson LE, Mazurak VC. N-3 polyunsaturated fatty acids: relationship to inflammation in healthy adults and adults exhibiting features of metabolic syndrome. *Lipids.* 2013;48(4):319-332. doi:10.1007/s11745-013-3774-6. https://pubmed.ncbi.nlm.nih.gov/23456976/.

25. Grey, Andrew, and Bolland, Mark. "Clinical Trial Evidence and Use of Fish Oil Supplements." *JAMA Intern Med.* 2014;174(3):460-462. doi:10.1001/jamainternmed.2013.12765. https://jamanetwork.com/journals/jamainternalmedicine/fullarticle/1787690.

26. Rizza S, Tesauro M, Cardillo C, et al. Fish oil supplementation improves endothelial function in normoglycemic offspring of patients with type 2 diabetes. *Atherosclerosis.* 2009;206(2):569-574. doi:10.1016/j.atherosclerosis.2009.03.006. https://www.ncbi.nlm.nih.gov/pubmed/19394939.

27. Ciubotaru I, Lee YS, Wander RC. Dietary fish oil decreases C-reactive protein, interleukin-6, and triacylglycerol to HDL-cholesterol ratio in postmenopausal women on HRT. *J Nutr Biochem.* 2003;14(9):513-521. doi:10.1016/s0955-2863(03)00101-3. https://www.ncbi.nlm.nih.gov/pubmed/14505813.

28. Warner JG Jr, Ullrich IH, Albrink MJ, Yeater RA. Combined effects of aerobic exercise and omega-3 fatty acids in

hyperlipidemic persons. *Med Sci Sports Exerc.* 1989;21(5):498-505. https://www.ncbi.nlm.nih.gov/pubmed/2691812.

29. Bernstein AM, Ding EL, Willett WC, Rimm EB. A meta-analysis shows that docosahexaenoic acid from algal oil reduces serum triglycerides and increases HDL-cholesterol and LDL-cholesterol in persons without coronary heart disease. *J Nutr.* 2012;142(1):99-104. doi:10.3945/jn.111.148973. https://www.ncbi.nlm.nih.gov/pubmed/22113870.

30. Eslick GD, Howe PR, Smith C, Priest R, Bensoussan A. Benefits of fish oil supplementation in hyperlipidemia: a systematic review and meta-analysis. *Int J Cardiol.* 2009;136(1):4-16. doi:10.1016/j.ijcard.2008.03.092.. https://www.ncbi.nlm.nih.gov/pubmed/18774613.

31. Ramel A, Martinez JA, Kiely M, Bandarra NM, Thorsdottir I. Moderate consumption of fatty fish reduces diastolic blood pressure in overweight and obese European young adults during energy restriction. *Nutrition.* 2010;26(2):168-174. doi:10.1016/j.nut.2009.04.002. https://www.ncbi.nlm.nih.gov/pubmed/19487105.

32. Shidfar F, Keshavarz A, Hosseyni S, Ameri A, Yarahmadi S. Effects of omega-3 fatty acid supplements on serum lipids, apolipoproteins and malondialdehyde in type 2 diabetes patients. *East Mediterr Health J.* 2008;14(2):305-313. https://www.ncbi.nlm.nih.gov/pubmed/18561722.

33. Dewailly E, Blanchet C, Gingras S, Lemieux S, Holub BJ. Fish consumption and blood lipids in three ethnic groups of Québec (Canada). *Lipids.* 2003;38(4):359-365. doi:10.1007/s11745-003-1070-4. https://www.ncbi.nlm.nih.gov/pubmed/12848280.

34. SanGiovanni JP, Chew EY. The role of omega-3 long-chain polyunsaturated fatty acids in health and disease of the retina. *Prog Retin Eye Res.* 2005;24(1):87-138. doi:10.1016/j.preteyeres.2004.06.002. https://www.ncbi.nlm.nih.gov/pubmed/15555528.

35. Shima Jazayeri, Mehdi Tehrani-Doost, Seyed A. Keshavarz, Mostafa Hosseini, Abolghassem Djazayery, Homayoun Amini, Mahmoud Jalali & Malcolm Peet (2008) Comparison of therapeutic effects of omega-3 fatty acid eicosapentaenoic acid and fluoxetine, separately and in combination, in major depressive disorder, *Australian and New Zealand Journal of Psychiatry*, 42:3, 192-198, DOI: 10.1080/00048670701827275. https://www.tandfonline.com/doi/abs/10.1080/00048670701827

275.

36. Kiecolt-Glaser JK, Belury MA, Andridge R, Malarkey WB, Glaser R. Omega-3 supplementation lowers inflammation and anxiety in medical students: a randomized controlled trial. *Brain Behav Immun.* 2011;25(8):1725-1734. doi:10.1016/j.bbi.2011.07.229. https://www.ncbi.nlm.nih.gov/pubmed/21784145.

37. Ginty, Annie T. and Conklin, Sarah M. "Short-term supplementation of acute long-chain omega-3 polyunsaturated fatty acids may alter depression status and decrease symptomology among young adults with depression: A preliminary randomized and placebo controlled trial." *Psychiatry Research.* Volume 229, Issues 1–2, 30 September 2015, Pages 485-489. https://www.sciencedirect.com/science/article/abs/pii/S016517811 5003844.

38. Lin PY, Su KP. A meta-analytic review of double-blind, placebo-controlled trials of antidepressant efficacy of omega-3 fatty acids. *J Clin Psychiatry.* 2007;68(7):1056-1061. doi:10.4088/jcp.v68n0712. https://www.ncbi.nlm.nih.gov/pubmed/17685742.

39. "Lingonberry Seed Oil." *NatureInABottle.com.* https://www.natureinbottle.com/product/lingonberry_seed_oil

40. Matsumoto, Takumi. *Phytochemistry Research Progress.* Nova Publishers, 2008.

41. He-ci Yu, Kenichi Kosuna, Megumi Haga. *Perilla: The Genus Perilla.* CRC Press, Nov 21, 1997.

42. Wszelaki, Magdalena. "How to Use Safe Fish Oils to Balance Your Hormones and Reduce Inflammation." *Hormones & Balance.* https://hormonesbalance.com/articles/fish-oil-omega-3s-balance -hormones-reduce-inflammation/.

43. Northrup, Christiane. *The Wisdom of Menopause.* Bantam Books, 2001.

44. Parker, Naomi. "The Importance of Omega-3s for Hormone Balance" *HoltraCeuticals.* https://www.holtraceuticals.com/the-importance-of-omega-3s-for-hormone-balance/.

45. James, Mary. "Omega-3 fatty acids—essential to health and happiness." *Women's Health Network.* https://www.womenshealthnetwork.com/nutrition/omega-3 fatty-acids-benefits.aspx.

Chapter 5

1. "How exercise helps balance hormones." *Piedmont Healthcare.*

https://www.piedmont.org/living-better/how-exercise-helps-balance-hormones.

2. Perez, Sarah. "U.S. adults now spend nearly 6 hours per day watching video." *TechCrunch.* https://techcrunch.com/2018/07/31/u-s-adults-now-spend-nearly-6-hours-per-day-watching-video/.

3. Marcin, Ashley. "What Are the Benefits of Aerobic Exercise?" *Healthline.* https://www.healthline.com/health/fitness-exercise/benefits-of-aerobic-exercise.

Chapter 6

1. Leproult, Rachel and Cauter, Eve Van. "Role of Sleep and Sleep Loss in Hormonal Release and Metabolism." *Endocr Dev.* Author manuscript; available in PMC 2011 Mar 28. Published in final edited form as: Endocr Dev. 2010; 17: 11–21. Published online 2009 Nov 24. doi: 10.1159/000262524. https://www.ncbi.nlm.nih.gov/pmc/articles/PMC3065172/.

2. Watson, Stephanie and Cherney, Kristeen. "The Effects of Sleep Deprivation on Your Body." *Healthline.* https://www.healthline.com/health/sleep-deprivation/effects-on-body.

3. "Sleep, Women and Heart Disease." *American Heart Association.* https://www.heart.org/en/healthy-living/go-red-get-fit/sleep-women-and-heart-disease.

4. Fotedar, Amita. "Sleep Deprivation: Symptoms, Effects, Treatments, & Prevention." *Sleep Standards.* https://sleepstandards.com/sleep-deprivation/#Sleep_Deprivation_%E2%80%93_Effects.

5. Davis, Kathleen. "What to know about sleep deprivation." *Medical News Today.* https://www.medicalnewstoday.com/articles/307334#effects.

6. Hormone Health Network."Sleep and Circadian Rhythm | Endocrine Society." Hormone.org, Endocrine Society, 21 May 2020, https://www.hormone.org/your-health-and-hormones/sleep-and-circadian-rhythm.

7. Shaw, Gina. "Women, Hormones, and Sleep Problems." *WebMD.* https://www.webmd.com/sleep-disorders/features/women-hormones-sleep-problems#1.

8. "Cortisol." *You and Your Hormones.* Society for Endocrinology. https://www.yourhormones.info/hormones/cortisol.aspx.

9. Laura Fenster, Kirsten Waller, John Chen, Alan E. Hubbard, Gayle C. Windham, Eric Elkin, and Shanna Swan.

Psychological Stress in the Workplace and Menstrual Function. American Journal of Epidemiology. 1999;149:127-34.

10. Pick, Marcelle. "Stress and Hormones – How Stress Affects Your Hormonal Health." *MarcellePick.com.* https://marcellepick.com/stress-and-hormones/.

11. Gold, Iris. "Hormonal Health For Women: What's Stress Got to Do With It?" *Fullscript.* https://fullscript.com/blog/stress-effects-hormone-health-in-women.

About the Author

Kamili Kiongozi is a designer, entrepreneur, and a woman who believes in living the best life possible. She has lived in 7 countries, traveled to more than 20, and speaks 3 languages. Kamili has been a saleswoman, a teacher, a dive instructor, a researcher, a web developer, a graphic designer, and is currently a wine startup founder. When she's not researching new projects, she enjoys motorcycling, cooking, and planning new adventures.